YOUR KNOWLEDGE HAS VALUE

- We will publish your bachelor's and master's thesis, essays and papers

- Your own eBook and book - sold worldwide in all relevant shops

- Earn money with each sale

Upload your text at www.GRIN.com
and publish for free

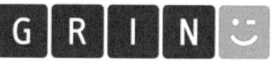

Bibliographic information published by the German National Library:

The German National Library lists this publication in the National Bibliography; detailed bibliographic data are available on the Internet at http://dnb.dnb.de .

This book is copyright material and must not be copied, reproduced, transferred, distributed, leased, licensed or publicly performed or used in any way except as specifically permitted in writing by the publishers, as allowed under the terms and conditions under which it was purchased or as strictly permitted by applicable copyright law. Any unauthorized distribution or use of this text may be a direct infringement of the author s and publisher s rights and those responsible may be liable in law accordingly.

Imprint:

Copyright © 2018 GRIN Verlag
Print and binding: Books on Demand GmbH, Norderstedt Germany
ISBN: 9783668642027

This book at GRIN:

https://www.grin.com/document/412258

Patrick Kimuyu

The Controversy Surrounding Affirmative Action

GRIN Verlag

GRIN - Your knowledge has value

Since its foundation in 1998, GRIN has specialized in publishing academic texts by students, college teachers and other academics as e-book and printed book. The website www.grin.com is an ideal platform for presenting term papers, final papers, scientific essays, dissertations and specialist books.

Visit us on the internet:

http://www.grin.com/

http://www.facebook.com/grincom

http://www.twitter.com/grin_com

Content

Abstract 2

Introduction 3

Affirmative Action Controversy 4

Arguments for Affirmative Action 5

Arguments against Affirmative Action 6

Women Status and Racial Minorities 6

Policy Alternatives 7

Recommendations on Policy 8

References 9

Abstract

Affirmative action refers to a policy that gives very special consideration to minority groups and women.

In retrospect, the controversy surrounding affirmative action is demonstrated by the divide in the judicial system regarding the justification of this policy perspective. Additionally, the public, policy makers and the international community express diverse perceptions on affirmative action.

Proponents of affirmative action argue that this policy promotes diversity and provide utilitarian justice to women and minority groups. In contrast, opponents observe that affirmative action undermines meritocracy, as well as perpetuating reverse discrimination.

Overall, women and minority groups are underrepresented in the workforce, as well as college admissions.

Alternatives such as socioeconomic affirmative action programs, including outreach programs, percent plans and extending financial aid to disadvantaged populations will enhance the achievement of gender, ethnic and racial equality.

Introduction

Affirmative action is a critical issue internally as well as externally the corridors of justice. Generally, affirmative action refers to a policy that gives very special consideration to minority groups and women. Eden and Ryan (2000) define affirmative action as "policies and practices meant to counter the effects of past racism and level the playing field in today's society" (par. 2). It simply means that the minorities are preferably admitted to schools or employed in government and businesses. By emphasizing on the problem, these minority groups will be assured of securing jobs and higher education. Through Affirmative action policies, proper actions will be taken. The actions will ensure that the minorities get job promotions, salary increases, career advancement, school admissions and financial support (Massey, 2004). Historically, the first idea of affirmative action was from President Franklin Roosevelt's New Deal that sought to counter the adverse consequences of the Great Depression (Terjesen & Sealy, 2016). However, the term had appeared in the Wagner Act, also known as the National Labor Relations Act of 1935 (Anderson, 2004). During this period, the United States was experiencing problems of proportions. To end these segregations, Roosevelt gave powerful executive orders that aimed at realizing equal treatment that failed to materialize. The orders were later coiled into Affirmative action under President John F. Kennedy's administration ("The Evolution of Affirmative Action," 2015). The research paper will discuss the controversy surrounding affirmative action and present the opposing views. Additionally, it will highlight the status of women and minorities. Finally, it will discuss policy alternatives and conclude with recommendations that would suggest better ways to come up with complementary programs.

Affirmative Action Controversy

In retrospect, the primary objective of affirmative action was to create equal opportunity to people, especially in the sectors of higher education and employment. Many nations worldwide now practice affirmative action in various organizations, but it remains a controversial issue with both positive and adverse effects (The Evolution of Affirmative Action, 2015; Terjesen & Sealy, 2016). The controversy surrounding affirmative action is demonstrated by the divide in the judicial system regarding the justification of this policy perspective. Additionally, the public, policy makers and the international community express diverse perceptions on affirmative action.

Of concern is the divide in the judicial system over the issue of affirmative action in which the Supreme Court appears to justify the approach from one perspective and denounce such justification from another perspective. Historically, affirmative action has always been contested in the judicial grounds. An outstanding example of this controversy is provided by the Fisher v. University of Texas which had been heard in 2012, but it has been sent back for further findings (de Vogue, 2015). Similar cases regarding the adoption of affirmative action policies in US universities had been decided in a non-consensus application of the law. For instance, the Supreme Court's ruling on the two exceptional cases in 2003; *Grutter v. Bollinger* [02-241] case and *Gratz v. Bollinger* [02-516] case demonstrates the old-age controversy in the interpretation of the law in relation to the legality of affirmative action policies and programs. Both cases challenged the constitutionality of the affirmative action admissions policy of the University of Michigan. In *Grutter v. Bollinger* case, the Supreme Court upheld the practice of affirmative action, which resonates within racial, ethnicity and gender inequalities, as constitutional (Pollak, 2005). However, the ruling in *Gratz v. Bollinger* case by the same court held that gender quotas or racial quotas for college admissions were unconstitutional (Perry, 2007). Overall, court rulings on different cases related to affirmative action have intensified the controversy surrounding the issue (Robinson, Seydel & Douglas, 1998). Therefore, it is quite surprising that there has never been consensus over the justification of affirmative action by the court system in the United States, as well as in other countries. In the one side, there are those who consider affirmative action as a justifiable way of providing social justice to the minority groups in the society through preferential treatment. This way, affirmative action levels the playing field through providing equality of opportunity in education and workforce. On the other side, opponents of affirmative action as a 'reverse discrimination,' especially from the perspective of equal treatment of all individuals irrespective of their social conditions, including race, ethnicity and gender. As such, they state that affirmative action seeks to provide historical compensation based on racial grounds; thus it is an unfair approach.

Arguments for Affirmative Action

One of the outstanding arguments for affirmative action centers within workplace diversity. Proponents of affirmative action hold that this policy approach promotes inclusion of historically excluded minorities in education and workplace settings. This argument has attracted immense concern in the academia, as well as in the political and workforce due to its implications to workplace diversity which has emerged as one of the main factors that underpin organizational competitive advantage. Card (2005) puts forth a convincing discussion on the significance of affirmative action as a tool for promoting workplace diversity in the business world. He argues that upholding the precepts of affirmative action demonstrates employers' acknowledgement of the role of diversity in the workplace setting in which individual differences are respected. As such, he observes that affirmative action promotes the creation of diverse workforce with talents from diverse populations; thus, enabling companies to gain increased competitiveness in the global economy. It is also argued that affirmative action provides an equal playing ground. Finally, proponents of affirmative action regard this approach as a way of counterbalancing historic inequalities, including exclusion from the workforce and education. In this context, it is regarded as utilitarian justice through which diverse association in learning institutions and reduced racial inequality promotes public welfare (Garrett, 2004).

Arguments against Affirmative Action

One of the most popular arguments by the opponents of affirmative action is that it is a reverse discrimination. Critics argue that affirmation action perpetuates racial and gender discrimination of those who are considered superior. For instance, it discriminates the whites and gives preference to other ethnic minorities such as the Australian aborigines and African Americans in the US. As such, this approach does not eradicate racial, ethnicity or gender discrimination in the global society. Second, it is argued that affirmative action reinforces racial stereotypes and stigmatization of the minorities (Sun Young, Pitesa, Thau & Pillutla, 2015). Finally, opponents of affirmative action claim that it undermines meritocracy (Alon & Marta, 2007). The principle of merit holds that equality of opportunity plays positive roles in the society. As such, it is claimed that the absence of equality of opportunity in the society may lead to negative economic consequences, especially due to the employment of less competent individuals from the minorities.

Women Status and Racial Minorities

Historically, women have always been underrepresented in education and workforce due to the notion that they are suited for household chores. In the US workforce, gender inequality persists despite legislative approaches to ensure equal treatment. It is startling that women remain underpaid in which the US Census Bureau reports that for every dollar a man earns, a women makes 79 cents only (Inside Summer, 2016). The same situation appears in Australia where men earn 24% more than women (Ryan, 2015).

Racial inequality has also been witnessed in many countries. In the US, the unemployment gap has not changed for over four decades. Unemployment is higher among blacks than whites (Irwin, Miller & Sanger-Katz, 2014). In Australia, the Aborigines have suffered employment disadvantage over the past two decades. Employment among Aborigines accounts for only 26.5% compared to 76.4% of non-Indigenous population (Norris, 2001).

Policy Alternatives

In retrospect, race-based affirmative action programs have created public contestation leading to the banning of such policies in some federal states although these measures are considered to be consequential (Long, 2006). Additionally, these programs have achieved little, especially in promoting diversity in US colleges and universities. Bell (2016) reviewed the contribution of the One Florida plan and the Texas Top Ten percent policy in increasing college enrollment and retention of students from underrepresented populations and found little achievement. This implies that there is need for alternatives which will increase diversity and retention without racial implications.

In this context, it is apparent that socioeconomic affirmative action programs will enable women and minority groups to achieve equality (Makinen, 2015). Bell (2016) agrees with this approach and advocates for the adoption of programs that focus on providing financial aid to disadvantaged students from minority populations and instituting outreach programs. She also observes that banning legacy preferences will enhance racial diversity. Percent Plans are also considered an alternative to affirmative action (Chapa, 2005).

Recommendations on Policy

Given the controversy and challenges related to affirmative action, there are several recommendations that can maintain racial diversity in the workforce and education system. First, the implementation of the policy should focus on eliminating socioeconomic barriers through racial-neutral approaches to counter reverse discrimination. Second, there is need for a universal legal framework that ensures affirmative action programs promote racial diversity and retention in the workforce and education systems. Finally, governments should institute effective strategies for enhancing the implementation of affirmative action based on merit and utilitarian approaches.

References

Alon, S., & Marta, T. (2007). Diversity, opportunity, and the shifting meritocracy in higher education. *American Sociological Review, 72*, 487-511.

Anderson, T. H. (2004). *The pursuit of fairness: a history of affirmative action.* New York, NY: Oxford University Press.

Bell, E. (2016). Alternative affirmative action: evaluating diversity at flagship universities under race blind admissions. *Ramapo Journal of Law & Society.* Retrieved from http://www.ramapo.edu/law-journal/thesis/alternative-affirmative-action-evaluating-diversity-at-flagship-universities-under-race-blind-admissions/

Card, R. F. (2005). Making sense of the diversity-based legal argument for affirmative action. Public Affairs Quarterly. University of Illinois Press via *JSTOR, 19*(1), 11–24.

Chapa, J. (2005). Affirmative action and percent plans as alternatives for increasing successful participation of minorities in higher education. *The Journal of Hispanic Higher Education, 4*(3), 181-196.

De Vogue, A. (2015, December 9). Supreme Court divided in University of Texas affirmative action case. *CNN.* Retrieved from http://edition.cnn.com/2015/12/09/politics/affirmative-action-supreme-court-university-of-texas/

Eden, J. M., & Ryan, J. P. (2000). *Affirmative action: contentious ideas and controversial practices.* Retrieved from http://www.socialstudies.org/system/files/publications/se/6302/630210.html

Garrett, J. (2004). *Discrimination and affirmative action.* Retrieved from http://people.wku.edu/jan.garrett/ethics/discaffi.htm

Inside Summer (2016). Gender inequality and women in the workplace. Retrieved from https://www.summer.harvard.edu/inside-summer/gender-inequality-women-workplace

Irwin, N., Miller, C. C., & Sanger-Katz, M. (2014, August 16). America's racial divide, charted. *New York Times*. Retrieved from http://www.nytimes.com/2014/08/20/upshot/americas-racial-divide-charted.html?_r=0

Long, M. C. (2006). Race and college admissions: an alternative to affirmative action? *The Review of Economic and Statistics, 86*(4), 1020-1033.

Makinen, E. (2015). *Achieving diversity: alternatives to race-based affirmative action programs*. Retrieved from http://www.luc.edu/media/lucedu/law/centers/childlaw/childed/pdfs/2015studentpapers/Makinen.pdf

Massey, G. (2004). Thinking about affirmative action: arguments supporting preferential policies. *Review of Policy Research, 21*(6), 783-797. doi:10.1111/j.1541-1338.2004.00108.x

Norris, R. (2001). Australian indigenous employment disadvantage: What, why and where to from here? *Journal of Economic and Social Policy, 5*(2), 1-25. Retrieved from http://epubs.scu.edu.au/cgi/viewcontent.cgi?article=1015&context=jesp

Perry, B. A. (2007). *The Michigan affirmative action cases*. Lawrence, KS: University Press of Kansas.

Pollak, L. H. (2005). Race, law & history: the Supreme Court from Dred Scott to Grutter v. Bollinger. *Dædalus, 134*(1), 29–41. doi:10.1162/0011526053124488.

Robinson, R. K., Seydel, J., & Douglas, C. (1998). Affirmative action: the facts, the myths, and the future. *Employee Responsibilities & Rights Journal, 11*(2), 99-115.

Ryan, P. (2015, November 26). Gender inequality still rampant in Australian workplaces, pay gap remains high: report. *ABC News*. Retrieved from http://www.abc.net.au/news/2015-11-26/gender-inequality-still-rampant-in-australian-workplaces-report/6976452

Sun Young, L., Pitesa, M., Thau, S., & Pillutla, M. M. (2015). Discrimination in selection decisions: integrating stereotype fit and interdependence theories. *Academy Of Management Journal, 58*(3), 789-812.

Terjesen, S., & Sealy, R. (2016). Board gender quotas: exploring ethical tensions from a multi-theoretical perspective. *Business Ethics Quarterly, 26*(1), 23-65.

The Evolution of Affirmative Action: A Critical Review. (2015). *ASHE Higher Education Report, 41*(4), 1-20. doi:10.1002/aehe.20022

Wasson, G. P. (2004). *Affirmative action: equality or reverse discrimination?* (PhD Thesis. Liberty University, Lynchburg, VA). Retrieved from http://digitalcommons.liberty.edu/cgi/viewcontent.cgi?article=1148&context=honors

YOUR KNOWLEDGE HAS VALUE

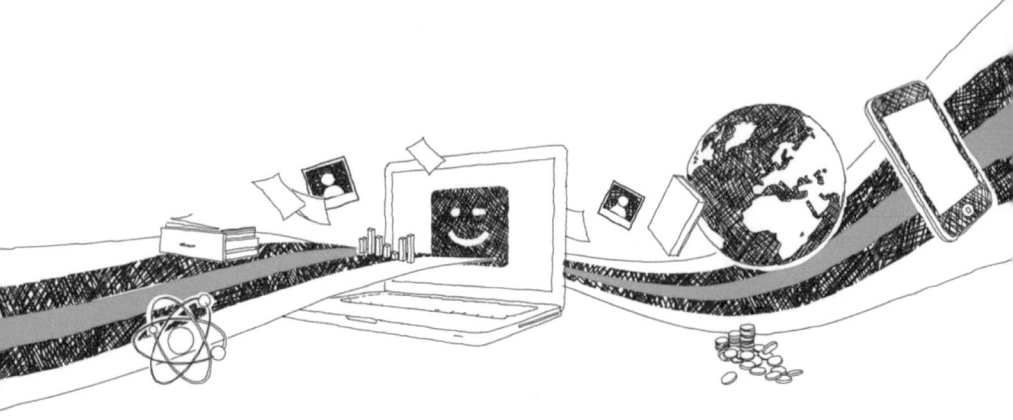

- We will publish your bachelor's and master's thesis, essays and papers

- Your own eBook and book - sold worldwide in all relevant shops

- Earn money with each sale

Upload your text at www.GRIN.com
and publish for free

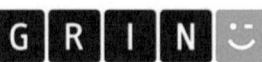